The Three H's: Hurting, Healing and Helping

By

Dana Y. Jackson

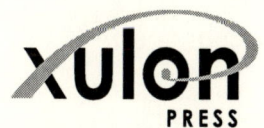

Copyright © 2010 by Dana Y. Jackson

The Three H's: Hurting, Healing and Helping
by Dana Y. Jackson

Printed in the United States of America

ISBN 9781609570125

All rights reserved solely by the author. The author guarantees all contents are original and do not infringe upon the legal rights of any other person or work. No part of this book may be reproduced in any form without the permission of the author. The views expressed in this book are not necessarily those of the publisher.

Unless otherwise indicated, Bible quotations are taken from The King James Version of the Bible; The Amplified Bible (Amp). Copyright © 1954, 1958, 1962, 1964, 1965, 1987 by The Lockman Foundation. Used by permission (www.Lockman.org); and The Holy Bible, New Living Translation (NLT). Copyright © 1996, 2004 by Tyndale House Publishers, Inc., Wheaton, Illinois 60189. Used by permission.

www.xulonpress.com

Acknowledgments

I thank my God first for pushing me into my destiny and purpose. Second, I thank my wonderful husband who encouraged me even when I was at my worst. Mother Jackson, your consistent prayers and life-changing words are much appreciated. Christina, Corrin and Destiny, I am grateful you put up with my hectic schedule. I love you! To Pastor Cook and Pastor McKelvey, thank you for sound biblical teaching.

With much love,
Dana Y. Jackson.

Table of Contents

Preface The Three H's ix

Introduction Spiritual Abortion xi

Part 1 Hurting 15

Chapter 1 Surviving the Hurt: I Think I Am Dying! 17

Chapter 2 Why Me? 27

Chapter 3 Embracing the Hurt: Yes, Lord 38

Part 2 Healing 55

Chapter 4 Help! I'm Stuck 68

Chapter 5 How Long, Lord? 84

Chapter 6 Light at the End of the Tunnel 89

The Three H's: Hurting, Healing and Helping

Part 3 Helping **91**

Chapter 7 What Now? 96

Chapter 8 Dispersing the Gifts 101

Chapter 9 You Can Do It! 105

Preface

The Three H's

Many years ago God gave me the title *Hurting, Healing and Helping*. I knew one day I would write a book with this theme. At the time I lacked the understanding. I was very excited and naive. I was also oblivious to the fact that deep hurt in my life would later cause this book to be birthed out of me.

Lots of times when we receive something from the Lord, particularly when we are young in ministry, we think it's for right then. Well, here we are ten years later. A lot has happened from the time God

The Three H's: Hurting, Healing and Helping

gave me that title until now. I have truly gone from a title to an experience.

Ultimately God wants His people to come out of the hurt realm and enter into their destiny and future. Unfortunately many times we are so badly wounded we don't know how to do this. This book will show you not only how to get past the hurt, but how to embrace it. As you embrace the hurt, healing will take place. For behind the hurt you will find a lesson, an experience and a promotion to a place you could never have reached with the ordinary life experience. God's design is that you fulfill your purpose. As you heal He will use you to help those struggling in the stages you just passed through.

Introduction

Spiritual Abortion

Most of us in today's society know what an abortion is. Whether through watching the news or knowing someone who has experienced one, we hear this word almost every day in our society. Merriam-Webster's dictionary defines abortion as: 1: the termination of a pregnancy after, accompanied by, resulting in, or closely followed by the death of the embryo or fetus: as a: spontaneous expulsion of a human fetus during the first twelve weeks of gestation—compare *miscarriage*. b: induced expulsion of a human fetus. From the Christians' biblical belief abortion is a sin. It was never God's intention for children to be aborted. (See Psalm 127:3-5; Isaiah 44:3, 54:13.)

In this introduction, however, I will be addressing spiritual abortion. So what is a spiritual abortion, and how can it occur? Spiritual abortion can occur when we willfully surrender what God has impregnated us with. We induce premature labor by rejecting what God has ordained for us to endure.

For example, maybe God is letting us know He's calling us to preach or teach the His Word. At the beginning stages we are excited. As we accept this call we notice that our families suddenly become stand-offish. We hear words like "holy roller" or "church fanatic." No longer are we invited to family functions because they fear we will point out inappropriate activities, such as drinking, cursing and so on, that are going on. Some of our brothers and sisters in the church say things like, "Are you sure

The Three H's: Hurting, Healing and Helping

God called you to preach?" We sense the skepticism and laughter in their voice. This hurts even deeper because if anyone should be supportive it's your brothers and sisters in the Lord.

Finally the disappointment, hurt and negative remarks become detrimental to our emotional state. God begins to deal with us about separation, especially from negative influences. Suddenly we decide maybe being a preacher or teacher isn't worth this. After all it wasn't until we heard and accepted the call of preaching that we experienced adversity. We decide we will just be "good Christians" for the Lord.

This is an example of spiritual abortion. We allow hurt and pain to dictate our actions. Unless we get back on track we have spiritually altered our destiny and purpose. We could have been the next Noel Jones, Paula White or Joel Olsteen. We aborted because of the emotional hurt and the effects of it.

The Three H's: Hurting, Healing and Helping

It's time we make up our minds that we will suffer no more spiritual abortions. What God has for us is for us. Pregnancy is uncomfortable, and labor pains hurt. Yet know that out of the tears, struggle, opposition and pain your destiny and purpose are being achieved.

Part 1

Hurting

Chapter One

Surviving the Hurt
I Think I'm Dying!

I remember a time in my life when I felt as if I was dying. Sometimes we can experience something so hurtful and agonizing that at that moment we feel that we are literally dying. I can only describe it as a deep wrenching pain in the bottom of my belly that leaves me gasping for air. Unbelief, shock, disappointment and constant pain seem to be the underlying symptoms. I couldn't understand it, but I knew my spirit man was grieving, my inner emotions scarred and my mind confused. I had learned that a

The Three H's: Hurting, Healing and Helping

person I had trusted in leadership had gone astray in a very disturbing way. It was as if I were a sheep lying slain on the side of the road. This also included my family. I couldn't fathom how God would allow this to happen. I felt deceived, tricked and alone.

At that time the Lord uprooted my family from Long Island, New York, to another state, as if relocating were the only way healing could take place. We were now living in Northern New Jersey while my husband was working in Rockland County, New York.

Every morning at five o'clock I had to drive my husband up the Palisades Parkway to work because we had only one car and I needed it. I distinctly remember bundling up my kids in the car (our car had no heat) and driving him from exit 2 to exit 10. The ride between the exits seemed to be the longest of my life. The whole way there I cried. All my husband could do was console me. I was reeling from the fact that I was living in another state, away from my church, with no money and quite unsure of my spiritual destiny, still hurting because of what leadership had done to me. On the way back, though, my tears turned into prayers. I remember my prayers sounded pitiful and jumbled from inner turmoil.

Yet through it all I could feel the sweet hand of God. I cried out, "Lord, I think I'm dying!"

He seemed to say to me, "This too shall pass."

I spent the better part of the ride back home worshipping God, never fully understanding the pain.

Many times Satan tried to convince me to take my life or walk away from God, but it was through worship that I was able to survive the hurt and pain I felt. It was in the moments of worship I found relief, healing and restoration.

We have a saying in the church, "Worship works wonders." The Bible says in Psalm 16:11, "Thou wilt shew me the path of life: in thy presence is fullness of joy; at thy right hand there are pleasures for evermore."

As long as I stayed in His presence the enemy was kept at bay. It was as if pain was suspended and life became tolerable. The only thing that brought me through was worship.

Worship means to adore; to pay divine honors to; to reverence with supreme respect and veneration (Noah Webster's 1828 Dictionary of American English). We were created to worship God. In layman's terms we are telling God who He is to us. He is a provider, a way-maker, a healer, a friend, a spouse and so forth.

We may ask, How in times of hurt can we tell God these things? Answer: the fact that we are still breathing and in the land of the living is how we can tell God these things. The dead cannot talk, worship or reverence God. Worship allows us to survive the hurt, because as we go beyond our pain and give God what's due Him, He addresses our needs. As we worship He heals us, even those hidden areas we have forgotten about or struggle with.

Let's look at an example from the Bible. In 2 Samuel 12:15-24 we read about King David who had sinned before God. David was known to be a man after God's own heart. Yet somehow he allowed himself to get into a situation. The text talks about how David took another man's wife named Bathsheba and impregnated her in the process. In addition David tried to cover this up by ordering the assassination of her husband.

Shortly afterward, God pronounced judgment on the sins David had committed. The child he and Bathsheba conceived would die. In the beginning David was observed fasting and praying, for his child was sick. Yet once the child died he washed, anointed himself, changed his clothes and went to

The Three H's: Hurting, Healing and Helping

the house of the Lord and *worshipped*. That's right he *worshipped!*

If we read further, the passage says David went in to comfort his wife, and this results in her later conceiving a child. The Scriptures record that God loved the child. This is the true meaning of worship. Despite how it looks or feels we give God what's due Him.

If we can learn to worship in spite of our pain we will experience an anointing to press on. Although the text does not say it, I believe David thought of every promise God had made and showed him. He remembered all God had initially brought him through—from being a shepherd boy to being chased by his mentor King Saul. The baby was dead, but God was still in control. He remembered all that God had done and all He promised, and that is what I believe helped him to heal and move on. Notice God blessed *this* child. Could this be because the worship he poured out moved God to restoration?

There is work in worshipping. We are *willing* our flesh to obey despite how we feel emotionally, mentally or sometimes even physically. Maybe your car has been repossessed, house up for foreclosure, your child sick or your spouse despondent.

Some of you are probably asking, "And you want me to acknowledge God for who He is to me in the middle of all this?"

My answer is YES! We must *will* ourselves to worship in spite of our circumstances. Worship allows us to survive the hurt. Surviving means to remain alive or in existence. Worship in essence is our life preserver. When we are broken, hurt and confused worship works healing and preservation. For when we worship we are in the presence of God. The why or details of our situation at that moment are irrelevant. Surviving by whatever means necessary is what's important.

Through the tears and pain if we can muster up words of worship—who God is to us—we can become true survivors of the present discomfort and pain we are experiencing. Sometimes it's hard, but not impossible.

Here are six questions that have probably crossed all of our minds. As you read the questions take the time to ponder the Scripture passages I've listed. This will help you remember verses that will come to your aid in difficult times.

Short Questions and Answers

1. Who should worship God?

"Who shall not fear thee, O Lord, and glorify thy name? for thou only art holy: **for all nations shall come and worship before thee;** for thy judgments are made manifest" (Revelation 15:4).

2. What should I worship Him for?

"O come, let us worship and bow down: let us kneel before the Lord our maker. **For he is our God; and we are the people of his pasture, and the sheep of his hand**" (Psalm 95:6-7a).

3. Where should I worship Him?

"Exalt ye the Lord our God, and worship **at his footstool;** for he is holy" (Psalm 99:5).

[Author's note: Easton's Bible Dictionary: footstool: connected with a throne (2 Chronicles 9:18). Jehovah symbolically dwelt in the holy place between the cherubim above the ark of the covenant. The ark was his footstool (1Chronicles 28:2; Psalm 99:5, 132:7). And as heaven is God's throne, so **the earth is his footstool** (Psalm 110:1; Isaiah 66:1; Matthew 5:35).]

4. When should I worship God?

A psalm of David, when he changed his behavior before Abimelech, who drove him away, and he departed: "**I will bless the Lord at all times:** his praise shall continually be in my mouth" (Psalm 34:1).

5. Why should I worship God?

"Exalt the Lord our God, and worship at his holy hill; **for the Lord our God is holy**" (Psalm 99:9).

6. How should I worship God?

"God is a Spirit: and they that worship him must worship him **in spirit and in truth**" (John 4:24).

Chapter 2

Why Me?

So many times while we are traveling through life inexplicable things happen to us. Some things we comprehend, while others we let slide by. The one question every believer has probably thought of or asked God at one point is, "Why me?"

See if any of these prayers sound familiar to you. "God, why is this happening to me?" "What did I do?" "What did I not do?" "I don't understand—am I being punished?" As Christians we will go through some things, good and bad, right and wrong. What we must realize is that we as Christians are not exempt

The Three H's: Hurting, Healing and Helping

from bad things; but even through bad things God is with us. Psalm 37:23 says, "The steps of a good man are ordered by the Lord: and he delighteth in his way."

That means when you wake up in the morning, brush your teeth, take a shower, eat breakfast, get into your car to go to work and then have a flat, God knew. He knew the tire was low on air and would run out of air. Did He tell you about it? No. He let you go through your regular course of the morning. Did He care? Yes. The tire incident didn't cause a pileup or car crash, just a temporary inconvenience. That's how life is. We must go through some things, but it's all for a reason and purpose. Even though the unexpected occurs and we don't comprehend it we must remember that our steps are being calculated by God because ultimately God has our best interest at heart. He directs our steps because He delights, or takes pleasure, in us. We are His creation, and He

The Three H's: Hurting, Healing and Helping

is always considering us because He loves us and is faithful to His promises. (See Deuteronomy 7:9.)

In Jeremiah 1:5 we read, "Before I formed thee in the belly I knew thee; and before thou camest forth out of the womb I sanctified thee, and I ordained thee a prophet unto the nations."

Before time even existed God knew who we were going to be. The only one it was a secret to was us. When we came through our mother's womb we were born in sin and shaped in iniquity. We came in knowing nothing; but God had a plan for us from the beginning. Even when we thought we took a detour in life God fashioned that detour to ultimately get us to that place. That place was a place of destiny and purpose. Here are three points that will help put things in a better perspective.

The Three H's: Hurting, Healing and Helping

1. Everything happens for a reason—even if at the time we don't understand the reason.

I remember years ago I was attending college, and at that time in my life I was also a new mother. My husband, Cory, worked so I was in a position of getting up and taking my newborn baby to the babysitter before I headed off to college.

Well, one day I had a dream that I got into the car with my baby and drove around the corner and my car broke down. In the dream, when I turned the corner, the right axle of my car broke off. I woke up a little perturbed from the dream but soon forgot about it. A few days later I got up, put myself and my baby in the car, went around the corner and guess what happened? The right axle of my car snapped. I was frustrated, angry and upset, and I couldn't understand why God allowed this to happen. Then God reminded me of the dream.

My question still was, "Why did You let this happen to me, especially if You already knew?" The answer was that God was trying to bring me to a new level of knowing Him. Needless to say I never made it to school that day; but my car went in the shop and got fixed.

The lesson was twofold: 1) "Even in everyday life I, God, am with you." 2) Maintain your car. The great part was I was only around the corner. It was cold that day but a very short walk. Even in the most minute things God cares. He is truly directing our footsteps.

2. Why not you?

As Christians we must get it through our heads we are not exempt from hurting experiences. We will have some pain in this walk. Paul writes in 2 Corinthians 11 about this pain and affliction. He talks about being shipwrecked, beaten, robbed, hungry, cold, naked and left for dead. Jesus often talked about picking up our cross and bearing it, for to be a Christian is to be "like Christ." We as Christians know Christ suffered the greatest affliction of all, for He gave His life for us. Yet it pleased God, for God's ultimate will was being accomplished.

> Yet it pleased the Lord to bruise him; he hath put him to grief: when thou shalt make his soul an offering for sin, he shall see his seed, he shall prolong his days, and the pleasure of the Lord shall prosper in his hand (Isaiah 53:10).

We sing songs with lyrics such as "Try me and see; see if I will be completely Yours." I sometimes wonder if we know what we are singing. We are telling God what we are willing to do and go through, and somehow we think it's just words. We pray, "I'll

The Three H's: Hurting, Healing and Helping

serve You to the end." But do we know what we are praying? Matthew 12:36 says, "But I say unto you, that every idle word that men shall speak, they shall give account thereof in the day of judgment."

We may say, "If You do this, God, I will do that." But when we get what we want we don't always follow through. We tell ourselves God understands, but does He really? (See James 5:12; Ecclesiastes 5:4.)

When I first became an ordained minister I was young, excited and on fire for the Lord. I told Him, "I'll serve You to the end, Lord, for You are my God!"

Three months into being a minister my husband left, putting me in the single mother category; I lost my apartment; and my immediate family relationships were strained. Every night I cried myself to sleep, not understanding why this was happening to me. The one Scripture verse that came to mind was

The Three H's: Hurting, Healing and Helping

that God will never allow us to go through more than we can bear. Even in times of crisis we must lean on the Lord.

At one point my two-year-old daughter was very sick and in the hospital. They couldn't find what was wrong with her. She was hospitalized, and it looked as if she might die. Every night she spiked a fever of 106 to 107 degrees. The doctors were saying she should have been dead. I prayed and fasted, not understanding, why me? Yet the true question was, Why not me? Was I exempt because I was a minister? No. My daughter was sick. I didn't have a car. I took the train to church and preached and came back to the hospital. When I went to the hospital room my little daughter was singing, "Praise the Lord," from her crib bed. I looked up to heaven and began to cry. How could she sing this when she could die?

A few days later my pastor came to the hospital along with his associate minister, and all three of us prayed and laid hands on her. The next night her fever spiked one more time to 107 degrees. Then after that as quickly as the fever had come upon her it left. Why would God allow me to go through that? Why not me? My prayer was always, "Use me, Lord! I'll go, Lord."

The result was no longer did I say God was a healer just because I'd read it in the Bible; I now personally knew He was a healer.

The Word of God plus an experience—a trial or test—equals a greater anointing. A testimony without a test is pointless. I can now say to God, "Thanks for using me."

3. Trust God through your storm.

This is a point we have heard over and over. Many people ask how. We must learn to rely on the Lord. Proverbs 3:5, 6 says, "Trust in the Lord with all your heart and lean not on your own understanding; in all your ways acknowledge him and he will make your paths straight" (KJV). Our problem as Christians is that we don't like not being in the loop.

We are a people who must understand why. "God, why did fourteen people die in that train accident, and we are the only ones who lived?" "Lord, why did so many people die on 9/11?" Many of us fail to realize God is in control, and no matter how high we go spiritually we will never know all the whys to everything. If we did we would be striving to be on the same level as God. But we are not God! He knows the intricacies of everything, for in Genesis 1:1 we read, "In the beginning God created the heaven and the earth." The Bible refers to the earth being God's footstool.

The trick is knowing how to accept what God allows, and that's by trusting in Him. We must lean on God—not the arms of flesh or our own thinking (it's too confusing)—but God's deity. He is God. The

The Three H's: Hurting, Healing and Helping

Alpha and Omega, the beginning and the end, the first and the last. He is ultimately in control. Romans 8:28 says, "And we know that all things work together for good to them that love God, to them who are the called according to his purpose."

God is ordering our footsteps. As soon as we trust God we will find that the trial, testing, processing and hurting will get a little bit easier. For in the presence of the Lord is fullness of joy. Trusting God as we go through our storm is a true sign of faith. Then and only then can we rest in His presence and have the strength to endure everything that's designed to bring us to our purpose and destiny. Why you? Why not you! You can do all things through Christ who strengthens you (see Philippians 4:13). Endure as a good solider in the army of the Lord. You can do it!

Chapter 3

Embracing the Hurt
Yes, Lord!

How do I embrace hurt? you might reasonably ask. Or better yet, why? Pain is pain, and nothing about it feels good. But something about it is necessary. That's productivity. You must ask yourself, What is this pain producing?

For instance, we all know it takes nine months to have a baby. At the end of the nine months the hoped-for result is a healthy full-term baby. One step can't be avoided, however, and that's labor. Labor is no fun with or without medication. Yet somehow

The Three H's: Hurting, Healing and Helping

women manage to push through labor, because they know the end result is another life.

What current pain or hurt are you experiencing that God may eventually use to produce life? Maybe you had to let go of some friends, or you are having problems in your marriage. Maybe you've experienced some very bad "church hurt" or betrayal. Whatever it is, know that God is trying to produce a "Yes, Lord" out of you.

So then let's pose another question. Why would we embrace the hurt to continue the process? Why would I put one hand in the fire and use the other one to hold it there? Because God is molding and changing us through our submission, pain and endurance.

Here are three things a yes isn't.

1. A yes is not convenient.

It's convenient to give a thousand dollars when you have fifty thousand dollars, but it isn't convenient when all you have is a thousand dollars. God needs our obedience, not our money. It is not always convenient to be obedient. But just as we don't want a sometime-God, God doesn't want a sometime-people.

Let's look at another example. Your boss yells at you in front of a room of coworkers. Everything in you says to yell back, get indignant and defend yourself.

The Lord speaks to you and says, "Hold your peace."

You are embarrassed, angry and annoyed. Your flesh wants to fight, but your spirit man says, "Yes, Lord." Even though many times we may feel justified, God is looking for our response through words as well as actions to be a "Yes, Lord."

Let's look at Luke 22:39-46. It reads:

The Three H's: Hurting, Healing and Helping

And he came out, and went, as he was wont, to the mount of Olives; and his disciples also followed him. And when he was at the place, he said unto them, Pray that ye enter not into temptation. And he was withdrawn from them about a stone's cast, and kneeled down, and prayed, saying, Father, if thou be willing, remove this cup from me: nevertheless not my will, but thine, be done. And there appeared an angel unto him from heaven, strengthening him. And being in an agony he prayed more earnestly: and his sweat was as it were great drops of blood falling down to the ground. And when he rose up from prayer, and was come to his disciples, he found them sleeping for sorrow, and said unto them, Why sleep ye? rise and pray, lest ye enter into temptation.

Jesus knew what the future held for Him. That future included pain, which for any person would not be an enjoyable thought. He asked God to remove what He was about to go through. Three times He prayed this; yet we find He tells God, "Let Your will be done." The Scripture tells us that even in His state of heaviness Jesus prayed. Although He knew the end result of His persecution, He still battled with the human nature that existed. He could at that very moment call a legion of angels to rescue Him.

But what about you and me? I imagine that as Jesus prayed, He thought about each one of us who would be lost, for without Jesus' death there would be no remission of sin. We were Jesus' assignment.

What is God requiring us to say yes to that is not convenient? More important, whose destiny or salvation are we holding up because the yes is uncomfortable?

2. A yes is not inconsistent.

Out of what you're going through God wants a perpetual yes. Yes, when it hurts; yes, when it doesn't hurt. Yes, when I understand; yes, when I don't understand. Remember that His ways are not our ways and His thoughts are not our thoughts. When you are financially broke or even homeless and God says to worship Him, can you stop and say, "Yes, Lord," and worship? When your car is repossessed and you're piecing money together to get to work and God says to sow an extra fifty in the offering tonight, can you say, "Yes Lord"? When God says to go minister words of encouragement to that sister or brother who stole from you, can you say, "Yes, Lord," and then go do it? We need a perpetual yes no matter what we are going through.

This is in essence what God is trying to produce out of us. Hebrews 10:23 says, "Let us hold fast the profession of our faith without wavering; (for he is faithful that promised)." If we walk in faith we will find that having a perpetual yes is not as hard. This means we must leave no room for doubt. No matter how bad the situation looks, even when it looks the opposite of what God has told us, we must trust in the Lord. Many of us Christians have become consistent at being inconsistent when we say yes. We must practice committing to a perpetual yes, not just in word, but also in deed. God is faithful. We must know this and believe!

3. A yes is not negotiable.

With God it is His way or the highway. What we must remember is that we choose salvation by our own free will. God will not make us serve Him. But out of our experience a yes will come, whether in six days, six months or even six years.

Let's reflect on Daniel 4:30-33.

The Three H's: Hurting, Healing and Helping

The king spake, and said, Is not this great Babylon, that I have built for the house of the kingdom by the might of my power, and for the honor of my majesty? While the word was in the king's mouth, there fell a voice from heaven, saying, O king Nebuchadnezzar, to thee it is spoken; the kingdom is departed from thee. The same hour was the thing fulfilled upon Nebuchadnezzar: and he was driven from men, and did eat grass as oxen, and his body was wet with the dew of heaven, till his hairs were grown like eagles' feathers, and his nails like birds' claws.

As you read the text a king took for granted all that God had done. The Bible says that for a period of time he grazed the field. The end result was that he acknowledged God with a yes. He extolled God and gave glory to Him, for He was God and creator of all things. King Nebuchadnezzar was told that a period of seven years would pass over until he understood that God ruled over all men and dispensed whatever He wanted and to whomever He wanted. After this we find King Nebuchadnezzar acknowledging God as the creator. He would never again try to negotiate concerning who was in control. When King Nebuchadnezzar said yes we find that more greatness was added to him. The end result was that he praised, extolled and honored God. God got a yes and a you-are-Lord-confession out of King Nebuchadnezzar.

Years ago I went through something that forced me to worship God. I was in a part of my life where I was believing God for some things and decided I needed to go on a twenty-one-day consecration/fast. The consecration/fast was going well. I wasn't working then so I was able to lie on my face and worship God, read His Word and pray.

The Three H's: Hurting, Healing and Helping

Day four into my consecration/fast a family member called. She asked how my transportation situation was going. At the time one of my vehicles was in the shop. We had a short conversation, and she asked me if I had gotten my Jeep out of the shop. I told her no. The bill to get it fixed was three thousand dollars, and I was still trying to gather all the funds.

She said something like it must be rough with only one vehicle.

I said, "I thank God because I still have another vehicle to maneuver around in."

"What did you say?" she asked me.

I repeated, "I thank God because I still have another vehicle to maneuver around in."

"Yeah, okay," she replied.

A few minutes later I left the house to go wash my car. I had just finished getting my car washed, pulled out and made a right turn. I then got into the left-hand turn lane. I was worshipping as I went and enjoying the day when I was hit by another car. I remember still hearing myself singing songs of worship while my car was lying there sideways. I was thinking, *Why is my car lying sideways?*

A police officer later told me he saw my car flipping over and over. They thought for sure I was dead. They used the jaws of life to cut me out. As they were cutting me out a firefighter crawled into the car to hold my neck steady. While the firefighter held my neck we had a light conversation while he explained to me that my car was totaled and I really shouldn't be alive.

"You're lucky, ma'am," he said.

"I'm blessed," I replied and told him God was with me. "Can I please get out of the car now?" I asked.

"You'll have to be patient," he said, "and wait for them to cut you out."

The Three H's: Hurting, Healing and Helping

I just wanted to get out and give God some praise in the middle of the street for saving my life again. I couldn't get out, but in my mind I praised God. I told the devil it would take more than that to steal away my praise. When I did get out of the car I praised my God. They took me to the hospital, and I was discharged the same day.

All that day people kept telling me I was lucky, and I kept saying, "No, I'm blessed." People kept asking me what happened and I relayed how I was worshipping when I got into the accident. This included the insurance people I contacted as well as the hospital staff—wherever I went. I came out with a scratch on my nose. God had in effect given me a mouthpiece to witness.

The next day I went to get the police report, and the officer at the desk asked if I was the one cut out of the car. He couldn't believe I was already out of the hospital. While I was there I shared my testimony with him and two other people in the police station; I also told my hairdresser and my friends and brothers and sisters in the Lord.

Day five of my consecration/fast I was a little sore physically from the accident but still feeling good spiritually. Day six my husband was rushed to the hospital with chest pains. He turned out to be all right, but the doctors gave him time off from work. His chest pains were attributed to stress. I was a little shaken but still holding it together. I brought the doctors' note to my husband's job. Day eight my husband called to verify they received the note. Day nine a coworker saw my husband's job posted up for bid. The supervisor at his job said "they thought" he had resigned. To make matters worse, my husband had no sick time. My husband called the supervisor, and he said it was a misunderstanding; it was straightened out.

The Three H's: Hurting, Healing and Helping

Day ten the nursing home my father was living in called to tell me that my father needed to go into hospice and I needed to fly to Florida as soon as possible.

Day ten I also called the police station to see if the police report was ready. I had been anxiously waiting, for I was told the police report gave an indication of whose fault the accident was. Upon reading the police report it appeared as if the report wasn't clear cut. I felt as if they were saying it was somehow my fault. I broke down and cried at that point. I no longer wanted to fast, pray or consecrate.

Throughout the day I worshipped through teary eyes. I slowly started coming off of my consecration/fast. It seemed as if I worshipped and prayed all day even though I still felt a sense of hopelessness. The truth be told, I was depressed.

My husband tried to encourage me to keep fasting, but I wanted to give up. On the way from picking him up at work in the rental car, I listened to a worship song on a CD. The devil reminded me that this was how I got into my first car accident—worshipping God. I continued to worship until I turned the CD off and got lost in my own worship.

My husband joined me, and we worshipped until the presence of the Lord came in the car. I felt strength and energy enter my spirit. I bowed my head in the car and surrendered my worship to God. My husband continued to worship God as well.

The difference was at this point of worship I was broken. This worship must have gone on for at least forty minutes. Even after we pulled up to the house we sat in the car worshipping. The presence of God was so real and tangible. I knew *then* that everything would be all right. He told me He was with me. God said He was going to give me a new anointing and take me to a higher level. "Trust Me, Dana." From

The Three H's: Hurting, Healing and Helping

that moment on I knew I would never be the same again.

Realize that even in your perceived failures, your hurt and your pain, God will still get the lesson through to you.

One day after the events had occurred I was thinking about all I had gone through. I asked the Lord why, and He reminded me I had prayed for this. *Huh?* I thought. God reminded me that a week or so before my car accident I had been talking with Him and I'd said it had been a long time since I'd witnessed. I asked God to give me an opportunity. In those two to three weeks I witnessed and testified more than I had since the year began. That wasn't the kind of opportunity I would have selected, but He did answer my prayer.

In addition I had also told the Lord my husband needed time off. He was exhausted mentally and physically from work. He wasn't eligible for a vacation for another seven months. God let me know He'd allowed the situation with my husband's chest to happen so He could not only deal with my husband spiritually but give him rest physically. My husband spent the whole week resting, worshipping, reading the Word and getting fresh instruction from God. Things that were confusing and troublesome to him became clear.

Many times we don't like or agree with God's methods. But no matter what happens God is still God, and He is still in control. He will never allow us to go through more than we can bear. We must fully say yes to the process even though it hurts. We can rest assured it is just for a season. As soon as we pass the test, God will promote us to the next level. We must simply say, "Yes, Lord!"

Part 2

Healing

Chapter 4

Help! I'm Stuck

What is healing? Webster's dictionary defines healing as 1) to restore to health and soundness; 2) to cure; 3) to set right; 4) to restore to spiritual wholeness; 5) to return to health.

If you see Sara in the mall and you want to hurt her physically because she hurt you or one of your children, you are not completely healed. If Johnny used to be your old boyfriend and he married someone else and five years later you are still up at night thinking about those past events with him, you're definitely not healed. So here is a million-dollar question.

Question 1: How do I begin to heal?

Answer: Start by being honest with yourself.

If you can never be honest with yourself, then who can you be honest with? In order for this to happen you may need to take an inventory check of yourself. So here's another question for you.

Question 2: What do I check for?

Answer: Hidden residue.

Hidden residue can be those things we think in our heads but definitely don't say out loud. I'll give you an example. When I first became a Christian, my husband and I thought the world of a certain individual in Christian leadership. For us, being new to Christ was like discovering gold. Everything was fresh and exciting.

One day I learned this individual wasn't leading the life he portrayed to my husband and me. Because

The Three H's: Hurting, Healing and Helping

he had been so influential in our spiritual development as well as being a close friend I was hurt and devastated. Eventually my husband and I moved to another state; upon the move I purposely lost contact with the individual. After a few years I told myself I was over what this individual had done and forgave them. Once in a while, though, I would run into a mutual friend who told me they had seen so-and-so. At the mention of that person's name anger and rage would simmer to the surface. Over a period of three years my anger finally turned to bitterness.

Well, one day I had a dream. I dreamed the rapture had taken place (see 1 Corinthians 15:51-58) and I was going to hell. In the dream I asked God why I was going to hell. He simply said, "Because you harbored unforgiveness in your heart." Hurt had finally turned into bitterness, and bitterness had turned into unforgiveness. In the dream it felt so real. When I woke up I was so happy it was only a dream that I wanted to cry. God had warned me that unless I changed my heart I was on my way to hell. The danger about hurting is that it can fester into something worse.

When we forgive it is simply to pardon someone or excuse that person from something he or she has done. We should recognize as Christian believers that all have sinned.

Let's examine Romans 3:23. "For all have sinned, and come short of the glory of God." In the New Living Translation of the Bible we read, "For everyone has sinned; we all fall short of God's glorious standard."

We must recognize that everyone makes mistakes, has faults and simply messes up. Some people have an ongoing pattern of willfully committing sin without a heart to change. We especially need to pray for them. Mark 11:25-26 says, "And when ye stand praying, forgive, if ye have ought against any: that

The Three H's: Hurting, Healing and Helping

your Father also which is in heaven may forgive you your trespasses."

In a nutshell if we want God to forgive us we must forgive others.

Finally we must remember that we must forgive with love. God said He draws us with lovingkindness (see Jeremiah 31:3). We must remember God is love. You can't heal properly unless it's with love.

Many of you might be thinking, "You don't know what Bob or Jane did to me."

The truth is, I don't. But what I do know is that Jesus forgave even when it was painful. In Luke 23:34 Jesus makes one simple statement: "Forgive them for they know not what they do." This powerful example shows the love we are to have despite the worst circumstances. I don't know what you think, but death is not a happy event. Jesus knew that these people were about to gamble for His clothes, hang Him on a cross and ridicule Him. Jesus knew what

The Three H's: Hurting, Healing and Helping

was coming, but He still forgave. The people at the crucifixion accused Him, spit on Him, lied about Him and watched Him hang from a cross. Many of these were the same people He healed, ate with, encouraged and overall ministered to. Jesus forgave us and forgives us each day; so must we.

If we are still having trouble forgiving, our prayer should be, "Lord, help me forgive. Please soften my heart." This may not happen overnight, but it is necessary. Through continual prayer and meditation on the Word of God and a release of self-will, God will help you forgive as you strive to walk in love.

Here are some correlating Scripture passages to ponder: Matthew 5:44-45, 6:14; Luke 6:35-38.

Question 3: What if that person hurts me multiple times? How many times do I forgive?
Answer: Seventy times seven.

The Three H's: Hurting, Healing and Helping

Matthew 18:22 reads, "Jesus saith unto him, I say not unto thee, until seven times: but until seventy times seven." So what does this mean? Your forgiveness is in essence endless as Christ's forgiveness is endless. But God has also given us wisdom. Don't let yourself be a doormat either. There's a saying, "Shame me once; shame on you. Shame me twice; shame on me." Recognize this person's behavior and proceed with caution next time, not holding the offense against them, but taking things with a grain of salt.

Let's look at an example. Aunt Betsy is known to tell lies. Let's say she told you she saw your spouse with someone they shouldn't have been with. You confront your spouse and find out it isn't true. You confront Aunt Betsy, and she says the person she saw looked like your spouse. Forgive Aunt Betsy for the offense, but next time don't run to the bank to cash the check so quickly. In another words until Aunt Betsy gets delivered from lying proceed with caution.

Let's examine another example in Acts 7:59-60. "While they were stoning him, Stephen prayed, Lord Jesus, receive my spirit. Then he fell on his knees and cried out, Lord, do not hold this sin against them. When he had said this, he fell asleep."

The Bible records that Stephen was full of the Holy Ghost. In the Holy Ghost are righteousness, joy and peace. Righteousness is simply doing the right thing. He forgave and prayed at the same time, for the Scripture clearly stated that he asked the Lord not to hold this sin against them. It was evident Stephen had the love of Christ and not lip service. How many of us can forgive in spite of undeserved physical persecution? This is where God is trying to get us.

When we were little and skinned our knees we had an open dirty cut. Mom usually cleaned it. She put on peroxide (almost every mom knew alcohol

The Three H's: Hurting, Healing and Helping

burned). After that she may have put on a little antibiotic ointment and a bandage. As a kid I couldn't wait for the cut to go away. It would be rough because the skin was missing, and honestly it was simply an ugly cut. In a day or so a clear patch came on then eventually a scab. Finally the scab fell off, and under it was new skin.

God wants to heal our cuts and bruises. In order to do this we must stop picking at the scab. When you pick at the scab you prolong the healing process. Not only that, but scarring and infection can occur.

Ask God to help you walk in the love of Christ. No matter how horrific the events are that you have experienced, God can help you.

Last, we must make sure we are not holding ourselves hostage. Maybe from the time you were five you knew you wanted to be a doctor. Thirty years later you're working at Wal-mart saying, "I should have been a doctor." Every day you wake up and say, "I hate my job. I hate my life."

I have news for you. Everyone has taken a wrong turn here and there in life. One of my favorite sayings is that it is never too late. Ask God to help you get a plan to pursue and endeavor. It will take time, but know this: with God all things are possible (Matthew 19:26).

Some of us have battled molestation, rape, past drug addiction and many, many other serious hurts. We may say, "I should have known. . . ." Or, "It's my fault, and if only I had. . . ." At this juncture these thoughts are irrelevant. The past is behind you. The future is in front of you. The most important thing is that you survived and are here to tell the story. Every time your mind or Satan tries to make you feel bad, recite these Scripture verses:

The Three H's: Hurting, Healing and Helping

Brethren, I count not myself to have apprehended: but this one thing I do, forgetting those things which are behind, and reaching forth unto those things which are before, I press toward the mark for the prize of the high calling of God in Christ Jesus (Philippians 3:13-14).

If you are looking back you can't press for what's ahead. God has good things ahead for you. Remember: "All things work together for good to them that love God, to them who are the called according to his purpose" (Romans 8:28). God loves you. Press on!

Chapter 5

How Long, Lord?

A common question is, How long will it take to heal? I would love to say sixty seconds or even sixty minutes. But the reality is healing can take sixty days, weeks, months or even years. The length of time is not as important as the method of healing.

The good part is that if you can recognize the part of the process you're in you have a chance of moving along and not getting stuck. Remember that healing is part of your process of development too.

God wants to heal you, but you must wait on it also. Ask yourself this question: What is God trying to get out of me? Nothing is by coincidence. God will take a situation and use it for His opportunity for three reasons: 1) to make Himself known; 2) to increase faith and patience; 3) to work on your character. How can God take such ugly painful situations and accomplish His agenda out of them?

Point 1. Getting to Know God

Let's look at Nahum 1:7. "The Lord is good, a stronghold in the day of trouble; and he knoweth them that trust in him." Psalm 37:39 says, "But the salvation of the righteous is of the Lord: he is their strength in the time of trouble." And Matthew 11:28 says, "Come unto me, all ye that labour and are heavy laden, and I will give you rest." Through the process of healing God will sustain you. He wants you to focus on Him, though, not on the length of time. For God is in time.

The Three H's: Hurting, Healing and Helping

In this next passage of Scripture we find an example of King Hezekiah experiencing sickness and having to allow God to heal him.

In those days was Hezekiah sick unto death. And Isaiah the prophet the son of Amoz came unto him, and said unto him, Thus saith the Lord, Set thine house in order: for thou shalt die, and not live. Then Hezekiah turned his face toward the wall, and prayed unto the Lord, and said, Remember now, O Lord, I beseech thee, how I have walked before thee in truth and with a perfect heart, and have done that which is good in thy sight. And Hezekiah wept sore (2 Kings 20:1-3).

The end result was Hezekiah knew with assurance that God was ready to save him. The text does not indicate how long he was sick, but we know it was significant enough to cause him to pray. Hezekiah was instructed by the prophet of God to set his house in order for he was going to die. God made Himself known to Hezekiah by healing him and delivering his kingdom and adding additional years to his life.

Now let's look at the second passage, John 9:1-3.

And as Jesus passed by, he saw a man which was blind from his birth. And his disciples asked him, saying, Master, who did sin, this man, or his parents, that he was born blind? Jesus answered, Neither hath this man sinned, nor his parents: but that the works of God should be made manifest in him.

For verse 3 the Amplified Bible reads,

> Jesus answered, It was not that this man or his parents sinned, but he was born blind in order that the workings of God should be manifested (displayed and illustrated) in him.

Sometimes your healing can take place in an open field. Everyone knew this man was blind from birth. Jesus told him to go wash in the pool of Siloam. (Siloam means sent.) Jesus sent him to be healed, for the Scripture says he came back seeing. The blindness was necessary and the duration of time even more necessary because it was living proof of his affliction. Maybe if he had been blind for only a few days or weeks a big noise might not have been made about the healing.

How many people have we encountered from the time we were born until now? So imagine that

The Three H's: Hurting, Healing and Helping

many people who know your lifelong condition yet now see your conversion? If you read further, verse eighteen goes on to say that the Pharisees summoned his parents. This miracle Jesus performed caused an uproar in the community because it was difficult to dispute.

Now let's try to imagine how this blind man was thinking and feeling. In verse six of the same chapter Jesus spit on the ground and made clay with the mud and saliva and then applied it to the man's eyes. After that He instructed him to walk to the pool of Siloam.

What went through this man's head as he walked down the street with mud on his eyes? I don't know what he was thinking, but I know I would be thinking, Is this a joke?

Imagine him walking. What's on the street? People. People watched the process of his healing. What did the people say? "Look at this blind beggar walking down the street with mud patties on his eyes. Not only is he blind and a beggar, but now he's crazy."

Could he have thought, I've been blind all my life—what do I have to lose?

The Scripture records he came back whole. His miraculous healing caused the Pharisees to summon him, and he acknowledged that his healing came from God.

Point 2. Increasing Your Faith and Patience

Earlier in the book I talked about when my daughter was sick and hospitalized for about two weeks. Truthfully it felt like the longest two weeks of my life. Two things came out of me during that painful, scary period. One was a faith that grew from a mustard seed to a full-grown tree. The second was patience.

Let's look at James 1:2-4.

The Three H's: Hurting, Healing and Helping

My brethren, count it all joy when ye fall into divers temptations; knowing this, that the trying of your faith worketh patience. But let patience have her perfect work, that ye may be perfect and entire, wanting nothing.

I struggled with the questions, Is God really a healer, and would He do it for me? That trial I went through gave me a front row seat to the healing power of the Lord. When I became weak waiting on the Lord I relied on the Scriptures. When my faith was tried it increased my patience. To do what? you might ask. Wait on the Lord!

I watched as they stuck my daughter with needles and tested her for cancer, HIV and whatever disease they thought could be causing her illness. The truth was they were clueless. Every test came back negative. The only thing that mattered, though, was that I knew my daughter would be healed. I didn't care

The Three H's: Hurting, Healing and Helping

about the method. It could have been by medicine or by miracle. I only knew that by Jesus Christ's stripes my daughter Christina was healed.

In your healing process you must rely on the faith you have. Every man is given a measure of faith (see Hebrews 12:3). Through your healing process God will stretch, increase and multiply your faith if you allow Him to. Don't kick against the pricks. Ask God to grace you with patience to endure the healing.

After you break an arm or leg, the doctor puts a cast on it. One indication the arm or leg is healing is that the skin itches. I've worked in the medical field and am amazed how many times people will try to put a hanger down their cast to scratch the itch. After a few weeks they get fidgety and want the cast off. Why? The patient is tired of being limited by the broken arm or leg. Some people have been known to try to break off the cast. If you can stand the process of healing the result is a whole arm or leg when the cast is removed. If you cannot stand that process, sometimes the cast has to be reset. That means more time out of commission. Know that out of your healing your level of trust in God and your level of patience will increase. Why? Because you are left to wait on God. Especially when man fails.

Point 3. Character Enhancement

The dictionary lists many definitions of what character is, but I like one I've heard a pastor often use when he preaches. Character is who we are when no one is around. Our character is to be "Christ like." Another definition is Christians manifesting the qualities or spirit of Christ.

As we are in the healing stages God will bring many things to light, simply by using the very situation we are in. As Christians we are supposed to bear the fruit of the Spirit. Notice that the Bible says fruit, not fruits. "But the fruit of the Spirit is love, joy, peace, longsuffering, gentleness, goodness, faith, meekness, temperance: against such there is no law" (Galatians 5:22-23).

We are to possess these attributes as Christians. If we truly belong to Christ it should be evident. Many times, however, through the trials of life our spiritual senses become dull. Healing will bring things to the surface, painful things, but it will yield change. As Christians we often fight against change because it's different and unfamiliar to us. But know that the God we serve uses many methods to help propel us to where we need to be. God will edify our character by fine tuning the fruit.

At a young age I had a pretty decent life. I never remember going hungry or being homeless or even sickly. The one thing I do remember is being a victim of molestation. For many years I battled with believing it was my fault and not understanding

The Three H's: Hurting, Healing and Helping

why it was happening to me. As a result I was a very angry, bitter child.

Eventually I told my parents about it, and they handled it the way any parent would—with a swiftness mixed with horror that this had happened to their daughter. I felt hurt, angry and guilty. Thus I, an angry, bitter child, grew up to be an angry, bitter adult.

As God would have it, I met up with the person who had molested me. I asked him why he did that to me. He gave me many excuses, but at that time I simply couldn't forgive or understand. On the outside I was a grown woman, but on the inside I was still that little girl who had been molested and violated. I was stuck in the hurting stage. I was like a time bomb waiting to explode. By twenty-one I was suicidal, depressed, promiscuous and living a dangerous life in general.

The Three H's: Hurting, Healing and Helping

One day I had a terrible car accident and almost died. About a week or two later a friend of mine had a similar car accident and died. Not too long after that I became a Christian. As God would have it He again had me see the individual who had molested me. This time the situation was different.

I had heard he was sick, and something in me wanted to see him for myself. I discovered he was very ill and had been told the chances of recovery were slim. He was fearful and confused and in agony.

The Lord began to speak through me, and my husband who was with me ministered words of life to him. I remember it as clear as if it were yesterday. We stood in his kitchen and prayed the prayer of faith. In our prayer we prayed for healing for him and began to thank God in advance for doing it. After we did he gave his life to God by confessing his sins and confessing that Jesus Christ was the Son of God who

The Three H's: Hurting, Healing and Helping

died on the cross and rose again. We hugged him, and within my heart I knew God had healed him; but I also knew I was healed too. I was set free. I truly forgave him for everything he had done to me. It was a very touching moment for me. Do you understand how long I had waited for this healing to take place? I had been molested off and on from the age of five to twelve. Finally at the age of twenty-one I was being emotionally healed. Forgiving him for what he did unleashed a healing that finally allowed the little girl inside me to grow up.

Lazarus, another good biblical example, spent three days in the tomb. I can imagine Mary and her sister asking, "What is taking Jesus so long? All the other times Jesus healed at the drop of a hat and performed many miracles. What about us?"

I want to encourage you that God has not forgotten about you. Just keep *trusting in the Lord*. He won't fail you. He loves you and has no desire to see you suffer. He wants to see you evolve into the "Christ like" person He desires you to be. If you can keep trusting in God and holding out you will see your expected end. Remember that no matter how long it takes to heal God will not fail you. Wait on the Lord and be of good courage. Wait on the Lord!

Helpful Scriptures

"And let us not be weary in well doing: for in due season we shall reap, if we faint not" (Galatians 6:9).

"Cast not away therefore your confidence, which hath great recompence of reward. For ye have need of patience, that, after ye have done the will of God, ye might receive the promise" (Hebrews 10:35-36).

"Let us hold fast the profession of our faith without wavering; (for he is faithful that promised)" (Hebrews 10:23).

"That ye be not slothful, but followers of them who through faith and patience inherit the promises" (Hebrews 6:12).

Chapter 6

Light at the End of the Tunnel

There is light at the end of the tunnel. Just as there is an entrance, there is also an exit. Believe it or not, this too shall pass. God is a holistic God. That means He wants to heal your mind and spirit as well as your body. When God heals, nothing is lacking. The physical, emotional and mental pain and anguish you may have experienced weren't for nothing. Your character has been strengthened, your faith increased and your relationship with God deepened. You in essence have lived to see another day.

The Three H's: Hurting, Healing and Helping

The very thing or things you have lived through have destroyed others. Some have committed suicide, but you made it and are making it. As you go through the healing process don't abandon the remedy. When we take an antibiotic the doctor gives us we usually start to feel better. Most of the time the doctor will give us instructions to keep taking the medication until it's gone, even if we start feeling better. Some of us stop taking the medicine. What is the result? A week later the infection is back.

Prayer and worship are essential to healing. Through prayer God will reveal areas we need to address, and through worship He will manifest himself to us on a greater level. In His presence is fullness of joy.

Many times when we are going through a heavy situation it feels as if all hell is against us. In our minds we want God to snap His fingers and bring us out of it. Yet if God did that we would not learn the lessons or reach the dimensions He had intended for us.

One day I battled with depression so badly I didn't know what to do. I knew prayer was the answer, but I couldn't get the words out to pray. A heaviness and a tormenting spirit hounded me. I tried to pray, and the words sounded unintelligible. I lifted my hands and began to worship God, and through tears I declared my love for Him. Slowly the pain dissipated, and I felt my senses returning.

I began to bind the enemy and declare and decree some things. God showed me clearly every evil spirit that was assigned to me, and I waged war in the spirit. I then went and laid hands on my husband and ministered words of encouragement to him.

Afterward I prayed and thanked God for taking me from *that* to *this*. What is *this?* you might ask. *This* is the place where you can now clearly hear

The Three H's: Hurting, Healing and Helping

from God and not from your emotions, demonic influences or confusion.

Tears are not a setback, but a release. It's okay to cry. Sometimes while God is working on us it's uncomfortable and hurts. Our tears are precious to God. Jesus cried. John 11:35 says, "Jesus wept." He may have cried for a multiple of reasons. Maybe for the fact that despite all the miracles He performed the Jews still didn't believe. Maybe because He read the hearts and thoughts of man, or maybe because Mary and other Jews wept. Whatever the reason, He wept. The key was He didn't keep weeping. He completed His assignment. He raised Lazarus from the dead. No matter what phase or season we are in we must remember the end result. The end result is that we are coming out on top *despite the pain.* Remember: "Weeping may endure for a night, but joy cometh in the morning" (Psalm 30:5).

The Three H's: Hurting, Healing and Helping

It's sort of like when we were kids and our parents took us to Great Adventure or Disney World. The sign read, "Fifty more miles." We kids got excited. Then maybe a sign read, "Five miles." Then we really got excited.

Can you imagine if our parents had seen that last sign and stopped driving?

"Mom, Dad, why did you stop driving?" we would cry from the back seat.

And they would say, "This is close enough."

We would have gone ballistic.

Even though you are not crying as much and things seem better and you see light at the end of the tunnel stay in the presence of God. Don't abandon what God has been doing. So if you have to cry, let it out. It is bringing you closer to the light. There is light at the end of the tunnel.

Part 3

Helping

Chapter 7

What Now?

How can all the hurt and pain I experienced amount to anything? What does it all mean? First know that everything happens for a reason. All you went through was not for you alone, but for others as well.

Hurting people hurt people. But healed people are qualified to help people. Help is to give aid or to assist. Be led by the Holy Spirit when an opportunity opens up to genuinely help someone through a deep hurt. If you have experienced the loss of a close relative this should give you insight regarding someone else's loss of a child or other relative. (This does not make you an expert, though.) Sensitivity and compassion should develop and increase out of your experience. Providing a shoulder to cry on or simply being there is a way to help. Prayer is also a big help. You may have struggled for words to pray while going through a trial, as I have, so you will have an idea what to pray for on their behalf as they go through a similar situation. Pray until something happens. Sometimes that means praying them through. They don't always have to know you're praying for them. But remember that the prayers of the righteous avail much (see James 5:16). There is power in prayer.

I had an opportunity to help someone who had not done much for me in my life. This individual was my father. My father left when I was two years old. He popped back on the radar when I was in my early twenties. When I met him then I was a Christian, and so was he; but I was still in that hurting stage. For many years I had wanted to meet my father, praying from the time I was a little girl that I would one day meet him. I realize now that at the time my heart was filled with bitterness, resentment and rage from his leaving and also from the events that transpired because of it. After a few brief reunions my father disappeared for several more years. My anger and hurt increased even more when this happened. Why did he bother to come back into my life only to leave again?

While my father was gone, God took me through several stages of development and healing. He taught me the true meaning of forgiveness and love. I yearned for my father, never accepting that at the time the Lord had allowed the separation. A few years later we were able to re-establish contact. This time he wasn't doing well, and I wanted to help him. He was a proud, stubborn man and refused my help.

This hurt me, but each step of the way I prayed for him, knowing God was still in control.

Sometimes people are unwilling to accept your help. The only help my father would accept was my prayers. Know that prayer helps. Finally he was able to get situated. We spoke on the phone because he lived far away, and I developed a relationship with him. For the first time I learned who he really was and discovered I had genuinely forgiven him.

A few months later I received a call that my father had had a stroke. The next few months were the hardest of my life, for at one point he was on life support. The doctors told me to make a decision on whether he was to stay on life support or not. I trusted God, and my father is still living today.

God let me meet my father and let everything happen the way it happened for such a time as this. God knew this time would come. I eventually had to put him in a nursing home and handle his financial and medical issues. He is doing much better. Now I can say that if God hadn't taken me through this process the way He did I might not have stepped up to the plate and taken the responsibility of caring for my father. Because I am healed I can help, and it's *effective help*. I can honestly say I am not harboring any ill feelings toward my father, and I continually pray for him. God wants you to take your hurt and pain and *help someone*. It may not be who you want it to be, but because you have been through the process you are now equipped to aid and assist people through the storms of life.

Chapter 8

Dispersing the Gifts

The pain you went through was not just for you, but for someone else. As I stated in an earlier chapter of this book I went through a very terrible situation of being molested. From the ages of five to twelve I was molested off and on. For years I thought it was my fault and I couldn't understand. I battled thoughts of suicide, depression, low self-esteem, sexual orientation and many countless scenarios.

I made it through everything. Reason number one was because God ordained me to make it. Reason number two was because someone prayed for me.

The Three H's: Hurting, Healing and Helping

God used me to pray and witness to the man who had abused me. God took my hurt, healed me and used me to help someone else.

Not only did God use me to win a soul to Christ, but when I forgave him for what he had done it released not only me, but also him. Remember healing is holistic with God—mind, body and spirit. When God heals you everything becomes renewed.

Since I have been saved God has used me to encourage many young girls and women who have been through similar trials. Remember that we overcome by the words of our testimony (see Revelation 12:11). I wasn't healed overnight, but I can now say I am healed and whole.

We are not to share everything with everyone. We need to use wisdom and discernment. But when it is time to share with someone share. Some of the mistakes you made may be avoidable and valuable to someone else as you share your testimony with them.

The Three H's: Hurting, Healing and Helping

We must learn to operate in our gifts. In 1 Corinthians the Bible talks about the gifts of the Spirit.

Volunteer. Moping around doesn't accomplish anything. Volunteers are needed everywhere. When you meet someone else's need God will continually meet yours. Look into organizations such as Meals on Wheels, Big Brothers or Big Sisters or consider being a mentor. An old AT&T commercial used to say, "Reach out and touch someone." There's plenty of work to do out in the world.

If you can't do any of these things, carry someone's groceries, give someone you know a ride or even sow a seed to a particular cause. Make a difference. That's what God wants. Take the focus off of you and put it on someone else. Walk in love.

Here are some correlating Scripture verses.

Give, and it shall be given unto you; good measure, pressed down, and shaken together, and running over, shall men give into your bosom. For with the same measure that ye mete withal it shall be measured to you again (Luke 6:38).

He that hath pity upon the poor lendeth unto the Lord; and that which he hath given will he pay him again (Proverbs 19:17).

For I was an hungred, and ye gave me meat: I was thirsty, and ye gave me drink: I was a stranger, and ye took me in: Naked, and ye clothed me: I was sick, and ye visited me: I was in prison, and ye came unto me. Then shall the righteous answer him, saying, Lord, when saw we thee an hungred, and fed thee? or thirsty, and gave thee drink? When saw we thee a stranger, and took thee in? or naked, and clothed thee? Or when saw we thee sick, or in prison, and came unto thee? And the king shall answer and say unto them, Verily

The Three H's: Hurting, Healing and Helping

I say unto you, Inasmuch as ye have done it unto one of the least of these my brethren, ye have done it unto me (Matthew 25:35-40).

Let us follow the example of Christ. Freely give and change people's lives through our testimony and the power of Christ. One word, prayer or hug of encouragement could mean the difference between life and death for someone. Disperse what God has given you through His healing power. Matthew 10:8b says, "Freely ye have received, freely give." You have received God's holistic divine healing. Now it's time to give back.

Chapter 9

You Can Do It!

So many times we feel as if we can't make it through the situations we are going through. What we must remember is that the devil, our adversary, doesn't want us to make it. His desire is that we die and never fulfill our destiny and purpose. God created us to fulfill an assignment. We have all been gifted to do something. It is our responsibility to find out what that gift is and move forward. Don't be moved by trials, tests or negative reports. These things will come, but always remember that God is with you.

Galatians 6:9 says, "Let us not be weary in well doing: for in due season we shall reap, if we faint not." Guess what? You are making it.

You are probably saying, "How do you know I'm making it?"

Simple. You didn't give up. The very fact that you are reading the last chapter of this book lets me know you're enduring. I'm here to tell you, you can do it. While I sat down to write this book I went through some of my greatest trials. Yet I still kept writing because I knew God had you in mind. I am here to tell you I made it and so can you. Through my storms someone else is getting help. Whether it's encouragement, strength or evidence of the power of God, *someone* is getting help. You can and will help someone too.

The Bible says that we overcome by the word of our testimony (see Revelation 12:11). You don't know whose marriage you may be saving or what

The Three H's: Hurting, Healing and Helping

young person you may be encouraging, but know *you can do it*. Whatever you are facing know that as long as you put God first He is with you. He loves you and cares for you.

God can do exceeding abundantly above all that we ask or think (see Ephesians 3:20). Trust God and know He is with you. Just keep standing and trusting in Him. Remember to put on the full armor of God and stand (see Ephesians 6:10-18). You can do it.

And now I leave you with these words. Fight the good fight of faith and stand! If you get weak and find yourself bending over remember that you might bend, but you won't break. And since you are bent over, why not worship? For in His presence is fullness of joy. We can do all things through Christ who strengthens us (see Philippians 4:13). Nothing is too hard for God (see Jeremiah 32:17). You can do it!!

Now, Father, I pray for every person reading this book. Father, whatever stage that person is in, whether it's in the hurting or in the process of healing or in helping someone, I pray encouragement and Holy Spirit boldness now in the name of Jesus. I bind the spirits of discouragement, anxiety and worry and call forth peace that passes understanding. Strengthen my brother and sister now from the crown of their heads to the sole of their feet. They need You! I thank You for doing it for them that they might bear a testimony and the ability to help someone else. Thank You, Lord! In Jesus' name I pray, amen.

Be encouraged! You can do it!

The Author

Dana Jackson is a wife and mother of three children and resides in Sugar Loaf, New York. An inspirational speaker, Dana is also passionate about ministering to young people, intercessory prayer and inspiring women from all walks of life. She is the founder of Women Be Inspired.Com, a women's inspirational resource. Her source of biblical inspiration is Philippians 4:13, "I can do all things through Christ which strengtheneth me."